Table of Contents

Gastrointestinal Symptoms During Pregnancy: A Comprehensive Guide

Gastrointestinal Symptoms During Pregnancy

1. Introduction to Gastrointestinal Symptoms in Pregnancy

A wide variation in the prevalence of the four most common upper GI symptoms, including vomiting, nausea, heartburn, and regurgitation, during pregnancy has been reported. It is estimated that 50% to 90% of women suffer from nausea and vomiting. A similar prevalence of heartburn has been found, but the duration of heartburn is longer than nausea and vomiting. Unlike other symptoms, there is a linear association of increasing prevalence of heartburn during pregnancy. In terms of lower GI disorders, about 20% to 18% of pregnant women experience constipation or hemorrhoids, respectively. Symptoms of constipation generally occur starting from the first trimester of gestation and increase as pregnancy proceeds. Recently, data showing an increased prevalence of constipation associated with a rectocele have also been reported. If left untreated, severe cases of rectocele can lead to fecal incontinence. Factors such as progesterone, which are also high during pregnancy, are thought to be responsible for a reduction in GI motility. However, an increase in pregnancy-related vascular pressure on the pelvic floor could also lead to the development of GI concomitant diseases. In regard to maternal and fetal health, it is not fully known what effect, if any, GI symptoms during pregnancy have. Several studies have shown that the hormonal changes occurring in pregnancy can cause exacerbation of a phenomenon commonly called "gut-brain" interaction, hormones that inhibit GI motility. Progesterone, which is important in maintaining a healthy pregnancy, can also cause symptoms such as GI dysfunction if it sits on the smooth muscle fibers and intestine property of the pelvic floor or on the same nerve cells. This could explain the close relationship between heartburn and constipation that is present during pregnancy. Accelerated GI transit also seems to be associated with vomiting in pregnancy and is thought to occur to reduce the likelihood of taking fetal toxins. However, the evidence supporting this theory is not clear.

Gastrointestinal (GI) symptoms are common during pregnancy. There are three main categories of symptoms, including nausea and vomiting, reflux or heartburn, and constipation. Gastrointestinal symptoms can start as early as a few weeks of gestation and may worsen as the pregnancy progresses. Moreover, multiple symptoms can coexist. It is important to understand the prevalence of GI symptoms, how symptoms can directly and indirectly impact pregnancy outcomes, and whether there are any appropriate treatments to ameliorate symptoms.

2. Physiological Changes in the Gastrointestinal Tract During Pregnancy

The alteration of digestive functions during pregnancy is related to various hormonal, neural, and mechanical processes. The plasma concentrations of cholecystokinin (CCK), gastrin, and secretin are significantly higher during pregnancy; this may be due to the decreasing effects of these required hormones during pregnancy or to an increase in the synthesis, release, or an inactive forgetting of one or more of these hormones. Marchbank et al. stated that the healthy pregnancy benefits women from a much-needed up-regulation of selective nutrients in the small intestine, which would lead to a corresponding up-regulation of small intestine function. The adaptive responses in the small intestine, and possibly elsewhere in the body, are likely to contribute to an enhanced availability of key nutrients during the gestation phase in anticipation of high fetal demand.

The research topic defines a relevant subject, which is referred to as a physiological adaptation in the gastrointestinal tract during pregnancy. This may explain the reason for gastrointestinal symptoms during this event. Pregnancy is a physiological event requiring various functional modifications of the woman's body. At the forefront, women experience digestive symptoms during pregnancy. Bloating, abdominal pain, flatulence, and heartburn were stated as the main discomforts by pregnant women. They affect the quality of life.

Gastrointestinal symptoms are usually due to mechanical changes in the digestive system, such as compression of the intestinal tract by the uterus, hormonal changes, a change in eating and psychosocial habits, and adherence to pregnancy. This document presents these different aspects and possibly their mechanisms.

3. Common Gastrointestinal Symptoms Experienced During Pregnancy

Constipation is bowel movements that are fewer than three times a week. Straining, lumpy or hard stool, and a sensation of incomplete evacuation are common symptoms of the gastrointestinal track. Constipation usually occurs when the food moves too slowly inside the digestive track. Furthermore, in the intestine, the water that the body has suctioned should into the stool can be reabsorbed, making the stool dry, hard, and difficult to eliminate. By the time that women are in the third trimester, physical and hormonal changes are causing delayed gastric emptying, an enlarged uterus pushes the intestines upward, and progesterone hormone relaxing the intestinal muscles all contribute to constipation. All of the above are reasons that contribute to the high percent of pregnant women that experience constipation. The hormones relaxin and progesterone, smooth muscle relaxation, reduce the motility of the gastrointestinal track. Lastly, women should be aware that late-term constipation could be an indicator of the development of hemorrhoids. Hemorrhoids occur when tensions arise in the area of the anus or rectum—they develop engorged blood vessels which can present as lumps around the rectal region. Furthermore, pregnancy also puts the new mother at risk to develop hemorrhoids. Hormonal changes that loosen and open the female pelvis in preparation for childbirth and the increased volume of blood during gestation are reasons pregnant women are at about to experience hemorrhoids.

Indigestion, also known as dyspepsia, is discomfort or pain in the upper abdomen. Women can experience indigestion at any point in pregnancy. Some of the symptoms of indigestion are heartburn, feeling extremely full after eating, a gnawing or burning pain in the stomach, bloating, and belching. In later stages of pregnancy, "gastrointestinal physiology changes: the pressure of the lower esophageal sphincter decreases, gastric emptying is delayed, and gastric contractility is reduced. These changes are related to the hormone progesterone, which decreases smooth muscle contractility." This change in the smooth muscle contraction of the gastrointestinal track is the culprit of most of the gastrointestinal symptoms experienced during pregnancy.

3.1. Nausea and Vomiting

Current research shows how deeply dysgeusia and hypergeusia have an effect on the mucosa. The participants primarily attributed the emergence of these sensitivities to pregnancy-specific hormonal changes with an average onset at 9 weeks of gestation. On average, each situation lasted for 12 weeks. The main complaint in the 3rd month occurred with difficulty putting something in his mouth, and all applications became visible after 4 months. For many women, new smell and taste sensations played an important role in food aversions, including an aversion to meat. Meat was the most popular food, with 16 out of 20 women stating that they now liked their steak cooked well-done, and there was no rare or interesting situation or risk.

Data also showed a relationship between the severity of chemosensory complaints and vomiting. Vomiting was found in 64% of patients with moderate severity, and in all (100%) cases of excessive severity nausea. Although nausea and vomiting are part of the physiological changes of pregnancy, mothers can experience significant discomfort and inconvenience, or life-threatening hours of suffering that affect the function of daily activities. Nausea and vomiting are a mucous membrane problem due to the very sensitive state of the expectant mother, and this also has a very bad effect on the fetal fat of the child in the womb. During pregnancy, food sensitivities are very noticeable. Table 2 presents 10 leading factors and details of chemosensory sensitivities.

Nausea and vomiting are mainly exacerbated by certain odors and by an empty stomach. More than half of the patients stated that certain odors, lots of odors (80 to 95%), and all odors (85 to 100%) trigger vomiting during the study.

Nausea and vomiting are among the most common complaints experienced during pregnancy, occurring in up to 50% of pregnant women, with the highest prevalence at around 8.5 weeks of pregnancy. Maternal progesterone and human chorionic gonadotropin (hCG) levels have been shown to peak at around 8-10 weeks, which is also the estimated time of maximum exacerbation of these complaints. The peak number of vomiting episodes was reported to occur between 9 and 10 weeks of pregnancy, whereas excessive salivation, heartburn, and constipation continued throughout the second and third trimesters.

3.2. Heartburn and Acid Reflux

Ironically, medications (antacids) of which the objective is to reduce this gastric acid secretion are the embodiment of symbolic action. The potential complications are insomnia, fatigue, hospitalization, c-section, lateral position imposed, frequency of diet, separation, and child depression. Anxiety is usually the most common trigger for gastroesophageal reflux, which particularly increases the impulses responsible for unlimited food intake in these women, and changes in microperistalsis. It therefore increases the usual volume of gastric residuals responsible for the sensation of reflux and/or gastroesophageal regurgitation, and therefore indicative of an increase in intra-gastric pressure. Providing information to the mother often motivates her to voluntarily stop behaving in a risky manner for her fetus. Allowing the arborization of the potential consequences of gastroesophageal reflux even wakes the desire to change lifestyles.

When heartburn and acid reflux are discussed in association with pregnant women, it is more commonly known as gastroesophageal reflux in the medical setting. These symptoms can present or worsen during pregnancy due to several causes such as the dilation of the uterus that pushes the stomach and the esophageal-cardiac junction up, increasing the chances of food returning back up, the reduction of the esophagus mobility, the progressive relaxation of the musculoskeletal part that is external to the gastroesophageal junction, and finally the effect of the gestational hormones which particularly relax general musculature. In one study, nearly 75% of women experienced this type of reflux during pregnancy, with a third pointing to eating as a trigger of reflux.

3.3. Constipation

One study that explored patient approaches to dealing with constipation in pregnancy reported that the majority of these women preferred self-care with over-the-counter options. Most of these women said they purchased some things to help with their constipation due to no harm and decided that if these items did not help, they would contact healthcare professionals. Additionally, some respondents testified that if going ahead with self-care with OTC options, non-pharmaceutical options would be an alternative taking into consideration that they would be pregnant. In some cultures, the use of the herb, Senna, has been documented as a common practice in managing pregnancy-related constipation. However, there was a rise in concern of health professionals in Thailand recommending senna for these women due to miscarriage. Moreover, before Senna was recommended to these women, some of the health professionals in the care of pregnant women were anxious to check with their senior staff.

Constipation was the most common gastrointestinal problem affecting pregnant women in this study. Although the exact cause of constipation in pregnancy might not be known, it was shown that some factors could predispose pregnant women to functional bowel changes. These contributing factors include women's age, pre-pregnancy weight, parity, changes in diet, dehydration, metallic supplementation, and lack of exercise. It was recommended in the study that constipation that fails to resolve with increased intake of fiber and fluids should be approached in a step-wise fashion using bulking agents or osmotic laxatives as first line prior to moving on to a trial of prokinetic agents. Furthermore, early recognition and management of this common problem will help in preventing the adverse effects of the condition on the quality of life of these women and their babies.

3.4. Diarrhea

Symptoms of diarrhea during pregnancy are the same as in the case of the nonpregnant person. And these conditions can also lead to harmful consequences, like dehydration. The fluid in a person with a normal body can be less than 11.5 liters, and compared to 15 liters in a nonpregnant woman or 3 men, the ten percent diminution in glutinous during pregnancy. There are only a couple of treatments. Therapy for pregnant women with diarrhea is advised to take the following seven measures. Diarrhea can result from any reason in the case of the hurting pregnant woman. It is also the case that the stability and water absorption have become more vulnerable, with gangrene rising by three times.

The most popular causes of diarrhea during pregnancy are: - Hormones (such as progesterone): During pregnancy, hormones tend to adjust the muscles of the cycling and the tissues all over the body, thereby affecting the function of the gastrointestinal system. - Poor eating habits result in diarrhea during pregnancy.

Women may have changes in gastrointestinal function, structure, and interaction during pregnancy. These pregnancy-induced changes may be of particular clinical importance when the patient has a pre-existing gastrointestinal disorder. Diarrhea is characterized by having frequent water and loose or liquid stools. It is one of the most common afflictions that are the principal complaints in a doctor's office. Symptoms of diarrhea can range from mild to severe. Colon disorders, irritable bowel syndrome, nerve disorder, and so on. Women are more likely hospitalized for diarrhea, and diarrhea has additional symptoms and has drugs to treat, like chemotherapy, antibiotics, or antacids, leading to nervous diarrhea. Approximately 40% of pregnant women have experienced diarrhea, and 40% have diarrhea during pregnancy.

4. Factors Contributing to Gastrointestinal Symptoms in Pregnancy

It appears that emotional factors either aggravate or cause stress, which could in turn exacerbate pre-existing symptoms. Gastrointestinal disorders exacerbated by stress during pregnancy are likely not a direct stress effect, but secondary to stress-worsened diet and lifestyle choices. There are other theories also to explain the etiology of GI symptoms during pregnancy, amongst which are dietary factors. During pregnancy, there are many changes in taste and smell sensitivities, dietary choices, and appetite. Decreasing the fat in the diet can help with GI motility and subsequent symptoms. Balanced protein and whole grain carbohydrates help with digestive regularity. It is recommended that 25–30 grams of fiber be consumed per day on a regular basis. Emotional factors, if already present during pregnancy, may worsen symptoms when changes in relation cause stress.

Like nausea or urinary symptoms, gastrointestinal symptoms in pregnancy are ascribed to hormonal changes. The most convincing proof in favor of a hormonal cause is that symptoms can be relieved when hormone levels drop. However, some authors argue that hormonal factors on their own cannot explain all the symptoms and that other factors have to play a role as well. In addition, the gestational hormonal changes also induce a number of physical alterations in the female body, which also affect the digestive system. This makes any symptomatology suffered by pregnant women even more diverse and complex. A study by Marsál noted that pregnant women at 40 weeks also showed an increase in gallbladder volume and the percentage of gallbladder emptying. These increases were greater in those women who complained of digestive disorders.

4.1. Hormonal Changes

The hormone most widely associated with pregnancy is human chorionic gonadotropin (hCG). The hormone responsible for preserving a pregnancy (i.e., corpus luteum-stimulating hormone) is generally elevated during gestation and high enough in the first few weeks of pregnancy to maintain elevated progesterone. Progesterone, a progestin that is distributed to the androgen fraction of hormone metabolism, appears to function in the form of an antiandrogen under standard metabolic situations. Androgens increase the production of substances that slow gastric emptying, while androgen metabolites have anti-emetic action. The shift in hormone metabolism towards increased androgen metabolism that results from increased progesterone during gestation may rely on a relative rise in androgens as progesterone levels rise, resulting in a potential androgenic effect in respect to gastrointestinal neurotransmitters.

As with many programs in the body, hormonal activity causes the changes that drive channeling of resources towards the developing fetus and the elimination of illness protective responses during pregnancy. Elevated or reduced hormonal activity also often underlies a variety of clinical symptoms, and it is probable that hormonal fluctuations during pregnancy are in part the basis for these physiological symptoms. Gastrointestinal motility, secretion, and absorption are all controlled by the activity of hormones. As a result of alterations in hormone activity as a result of a developing fetus, it is reasonable to assume that a significant portion of the physiological gastrointestinal symptoms that arise during pregnancy can be attributed to changes in gastrointestinal functions that are owing to altered hormone activity rather than the pregnant uterus.

4.2. Physical Changes in the Uterus and Abdomen

Considering these physiological and anatomical changes that affect the intestine, the metabolic and hormonal changes occurring during pregnancy can interact and potentially worsen if a pregnant woman already has a weakened or underlying gastrointestinal disease.

These changes can lead to various alterations in the digestive process. Taking all of these changes into account, we can understand why so many women experience heartburn during pregnancy. Moreover, although the most pronounced changes during pregnancy are changes in the hormonal balance and the physical hallmarks of pregnancy, such as an expanding uterus and abdomen, the functional adaptation in the gastrointestinal tract also plays a key indirect role in the development of symptoms.

Due to the growing baby pushing up into the abdominal cavity, the entire abdominal cavity expands to accommodate the child's growth. As the abdominal area expands, the movement of the abdominal muscles becomes weak and relaxed to accommodate the uterus and changes in the diaphragm and chest cavity. Consequently, the lower pressure that helps compress the food within the stomach and intestines is lost, resulting in an accumulation of gas and fluid in the stomach and intestines.

Physical changes in the uterus and abdomen during pregnancy are quite significant. One of the most noticeable changes is the growth of the uterus, which begins to increase during the first trimester. The uterus expands continuously, increasing the pressure on the surrounding organs, particularly the intestines. As a result, the intestines gradually become compressed, causing many women to experience constipation.

4.3. Dietary Factors

Special emphasis should be placed on this in view of the high prevalence of milk intolerance, functional milk intolerance, and/or allergy. All recommendations of dietary modifications are based on a low level of evidence and have direct implications for any preventive or management strategies. There are conflicting reports on the influence of changes in dietary habits during pregnancy. In a population-based study involving about 10,000 Norwegian women, "Westernization" of diet or adoption of an eating pattern characterized by low vegetables and high consumption of cakes and snacks might take some time before it became a risk factor for reflux; the overall association was limited. Moreover, the increased consumption of fruits, citrus fruits, fruit juices, sweets, soft drinks, high-fat and fried and spicy foods, chocolate, and whole milk-drinking, and an inverse trend for milk, white bread, vegetables, and low-fat dressings was only weakly predictive when eaten daily. In another large-scale study, the increased prevalence of heartburn and acid regurgitation during pregnancy was not associated with specific dietary habits such as the amount consumed and frequency of meals and drinks, consumption of fried food, high-fat food, onions, milk, alcohol, black pepper, tobacco, and dietary fiber. Thus, in a 24-hour period, food content may have an effect, but it should be consumed in larger quantities. It is important to remember that food will stay in your stomach. Short fasting has been shown to decrease acid production. With binding interrelated values to related food items in the liquid-solid/semi-solid phase and consumed frequently, and in smaller quantities, no correlations were reported.

4.3. Dietary Factors. Nutrition can have a significant effect on many functional gastrointestinal symptoms. As such, dietary factors may contribute to gastrointestinal symptoms of pregnancy. There is a close and complex relationship between diet and gut symptoms. A meal can provoke symptoms of gastroesophageal reflux, bloating, diarrhea, or constipation. Poor reports on dairy intake and lactose intolerance/suspected milk protein allergy were by far the most prevalent in our study.

4.4. Stress and Emotional Factors

There seems to be a relation between heartburn and emotional well-being, as well as the subject using any substance which modifies the state of the nervous system during pregnancy. During the last three months of pregnancy, subjects with heartburn took significantly more such substances (sedatives and hypnotics) than those without this symptom in pregnancy planning. It could be mentioned as a connection between bad emotional well-being and an elevated risk of heartburn in late pregnancy. Therapy of the condition could also be improved by psychotherapy. The connection between LUTS, reflux disease, and good psychic situation of the patients who suffer from them during pregnancy, as well as the disturbances in emotional health that accompany the conditions, should be further evaluated. All points in this sub-section are connected with papers by Jabłoński, M.J., Starczewski, A., Neubauer, K., Chudziński, Liticsa, R., Maciejewski, and T.

Stress is an emotional factor that may influence the sensation of heartburn during pregnancy, as well as the severity of the symptoms. The therapy of such conditions is always connected with the reduction of nervous tension. A disturbed emotional condition is often mentioned by female outpatients as a factor causing the intensification of these symptoms. Both the state and trait anxiety are suggested to be associated with a higher prevalence of bloating. Vazquez et al. reported that anxiety was the single most important factor affecting symptom reporting in pregnant women. However, in the study of Favaios et al., there were no significant changes between bloating prevalence and the trait anxiety scores.

5. Complications of Gastrointestinal Symptoms in Pregnancy

Fetuses whose mothers have long-lasting and severe dehydration or malnutrition are at an increased risk for premature birth and having malformations of the central nervous system, orofacial structures, extremities, and abdominal wall, and less frequently the heart and gastrointestinal system (especially esophageal atresia). Pregnant women may develop certain complications of severe and long-lasting nausea, plus vomiting similar to those of ketonuria. This condition is called "ketoacidosis" in the non-pregnant and "hyperemesis gravidarum" or "repeated prolonged vomiting of pregnancy" in pregnancy. Some women will develop ketosis and excrete ketone bodies in their urine before any physical signs or symptoms of ketosis appear. A licensed professional can measure urine ketones to determine when or how well they are hydrated and whether or not medical care is needed. Generally, if a woman does not or cannot eat for an extended period, she needs medical evaluation.

The 17th American College of Gastroenterology Monograph on Obstetrics summarizes some important complications that can result from nausea and vomiting during pregnancy. These are detailed in the section titled "Maternal Complications of Hyperemesis Gravidarum." Long-lasting gastrointestinal symptoms can lead to dehydration, weight loss, and imbalances in the levels of important minerals and salts in the blood. This can lead to complications for the mother and fetus.

5.1. Dehydration

What to do: If you suspect dehydration, try to keep track of the patient's fluid intake and loss. They should avoid diuretics because they can increase the risk of being dehydrated. Make sure they are drinking fluids throughout the day. Water is best, but adding citrus can help with nausea. Warm drinks or food may also cause less nausea. Small sips can help relieve bloating at the same time. Eating foods with high water content like fruits and vegetables or broth-based soups can help with hydration. For every episode of emesis or diarrhea, rehydrate with an oral rehydration solution. It is best to use one with less sugar and eat dry toast or crackers with it. If they are able to eat larger meals, encourage foods like rice, potatoes, gluten-free pasta, oatmeal, and iron-based foods. If the patient has ketones in her urine (positive urine test), then she has been fasting too long without eating. She needs to eat something small within 30 minutes or she will start breaking down her muscle to make glucose. If she can't eat anything, she should drink something with sugar like apple juice or lemon-lime soda to decrease her ketones; even a couple of small sips will help. If she is unable to decrease her ketones, seek medical care. If she is becoming dehydrated, she may need an IV.

Causes: Not being able to keep up with losses can lead to dehydration. If an expecting mom is dehydrated, not enough blood may get back to the uterus and can cause the baby's heart rate to change. This can also decrease blood flow to the mother's kidneys and cause problems there. It can even cause her to go into labor early. Dehydration makes constipation worse and can lead to symptoms like reduced urine output, dark urine, dry or sticky mouth, headache, and fatigue.

5.2. Weight Loss

EU literature and guidelines for clinical care of nausea and vomiting in pregnancy have recommended monitoring of maternal weight, with a degree of urgency linked to the woman's current BMI and her gestation. If vomiting that has led to weight loss worsens, the woman will become even more malnourished and dehydrated and so justify more clinical urgency. In addition, monitoring can ascertain if medications and dietary or social advice have been helpful, indicate something emotionally affecting their appetite, suggest a woman with very infrequent anti-nausea treatment might need another prescription between antenatal visits, or plan when a scan of fetal growth is indicated.

Despite the absence of vomiting, some women report weight loss during their pregnancy. Women with hyperemesis gravidarum were five times more likely to lose weight (3.4 kg; stop gain / weight loss: 4.8 kg) than women with normal pregnancies (0.5 kg, median increase in their first 20 wks)32. Nausea or vomiting occurring before 9 wks decreased the mean weight gain in kilograms in the first 20 wks in 866 reports from Sweden, England, and Australia33. The impacts of weight loss have been less well studied than the consequences of weight gain, but it is possible that the metabolism of pregnancy does prefer fat stores28, making fetal malnutrition the dominant effect of weight loss. The physiological changes of pregnancy may make symptoms less likely to cause unacceptably rapid weight loss. Many studies from the 1980s and earlier failed to observe "clinically significant" weight loss, probably because that proportion had already been "selected out" of the sample in their first months of pregnancy by the time their weight was taken.

5.3. Electrolyte Imbalance

Alterations in the levels of these electrolytes induce excitability changes in the physiological system, producing varying degrees of cellular disease and death. Clinically, the electrolyte imbalance comes into picture due to the increased load on the kidneys, causing tubulointerstitial damage and dysfunction of their reabsorption capacity. It is also shown that in these complicated states, metabolism might also be affected in the gastrointestinal cells, particularly in patients with irreversible and prolonged damage, and as an immediate effect of gastrectomy. A detailed study of the impact of electrolyte imbalance might provide further insight into the morbidity and mortality of pregnant cases undergoing this complication universally. This necessitates first understanding the normal levels of these electrolytes in normal pregnant cases and following cases suffering from unremarkable to severe gastrointestinal distress.

Having discussed the above impact of hyperemesis and resultant dehydration on pregnancy, it is now evident that vitals are not only a marker for the status of the patient but also reflect the health of her unborn child. An analysis of the impact of electrolyte imbalance in the body has the potential to unveil its impact on overall physiological changes in a pregnant woman. The electroneutrality between the cations and anions makes the overall charge in the body equal to zero. The major electrolytes are sodium (Na^+), potassium (K^+), calcium (Ca^{2+}), magnesium (Mg^{2+}), chloride (Cl^-), bicarbonate (HCO_3^-), phosphate (HPO_4^{2-}), and sulfate (SO_4^{2-}). Every electrolyte has a role. Na^+, K^+, and Cl^- are significant in the maintenance of membrane potentials, which are necessary for signal initiation, nerve conduction, muscle contraction, and the movement of solute carriers among cells.

6. Management and Treatment of Gastrointestinal Symptoms in Pregnancy

Quite a number of substances have been proven effective for gastrointestinal problems, including dietary fiber, low-FODMAP diet, prebiotics, probiotics, using fructose and promotion of relaxation, and co-therapy to alleviate their action. Some supplements were reported to adversely affect gastrointestinal functioning. Healthcare providers should counsel pregnant women to avoid these. Specific pharmacological management of IBS during pregnancy and lactation is described in detail in a further section. For women suffering from severe gastrointestinal symptoms, calcium carbonate could be considered over magnesium hydroxide or aluminium hydroxide-based antacids. All antacids should be used with caution in high doses, and pregnant women should be advised to avoid variable doses and to not exceed the manufacturer's guidelines.

The treatment of a pregnant woman has a need to change her lifestyle to improve gastrointestinal problems. Counsel regarding lifestyle measures and dietary changes is vital to improve gastrointestinal symptoms. Diet advice during pregnancy generally starts with relaxation techniques and peppermint, which possibly help manage heartburn and nausea in some women. Then probiotics or prebiotics, along with general dietary advice, are the next basic management level. For women with distract gastroesophageal reflux disease (GERD) or IBS, the basic treatment should start with the dietary advice listed above and treat them as separate conditions. Many general measures are available for the treatment of IBS and are summarized in Table 2. If they are still symptomatic, they might need a change of diet and lifestyle recommendations, addition of medication, or referral to a specialist.

6.1. Lifestyle Modifications

Rest: During the first trimester, up to 60% of pregnant women are observed to modify their lifestyle, often one of the factors that influences morning sickness the most. At times, they may need to alter their work schedule, rest, in consultation with their GP, or alternatively, change their work duties. In general, it is advisable to get enough rest and minimize stress. Not being able to rest or having personal problems may worsen stomach symptoms or favor the development of ongoing digestive disorders. Taking a real rest break also allows the resolution of dyspepsia and gastrointestinal symptoms influenced by tension, anxiety, insomnia, and the like. In general, reactivating the work activity before completion of the rest period may result in a higher incidence of gastrointestinal symptoms than those observed at the start. I'm sorry, I say signal with relief viable solution to psychosomatic of end. If the symptoms don't disappear completely during the holidays, they improve at least. It is not a dangerous symptom.

Activity: Although morning sickness is most common in the morning, eating patterns may also be affected, and these women may experience nausea at other times of the day on an empty stomach. Accordingly, it is advisable for pregnant women to have frequent, varied, and nutritionally balanced meals, decreasing the amount of food consumed and increasing the number of meals in the event of morning sickness. Caffeinated and acidic beverages, fried and spicy foods, and foods with a strong smell should be avoided. It is convenient to avoid going to bed after eating and to have dinner at least 2 to 3 hours before lying down. It is advisable to rise slowly and not to perform any sudden movements. Physical activity should be continued gently, avoiding physical overload. In the treatment of indigestion, the following hygienic-dietetic-digestive advice may be beneficial. A mild walk after dinner may be helpful, but rigorous daily morning exercises on an empty stomach should be avoided because of the risk of traumatic oesophagogastric reflux. We also advise patients to refrain from counting the steps after meals recommended to improve metabolic use of glucose by quotidian activity in type-2 diabetes, or therapeutic, as is suggested in association with a meal at bedtime in older type-2 diabetic patients.

6.2. Dietary Recommendations

Gastrointestinal symptoms, such as nausea, vomiting, and constipation, are common in pregnancy, with between 40% and 50% of pregnant women reporting these symptoms. Maternity healthcare should recommend mothers to avoid high carbohydrate intake, high-fat crisps, and prefer enough fluid intake and not to eat fiber foods. This recommendation decreases the symptoms of mothers and improves the quality of life. Fiber and fluids work together in the gastrointestinal tract to promote normal bowel function. Dietary fiber can relieve constipation, and pregnant women are recommended a daily intake of 28 g of dietary fiber. Proper care should be taken because if the fiber intake is increased very suddenly, it may cause malabsorption and other digestive problems, such as bloating and flatulence. Increasing the fiber content in one's diet may affect the amount of fluid one should drink; therefore, adequate fluid intake and presentation should be adjusted simultaneously with the fiber increase. It is important to have a balanced and varied diet, especially throughout pregnancy, as both the mother and baby also need enough nutrients. When the pregnancy continues, there is an increase in nutrient need both to support the mother's daily activities and to support the baby's development and growth. In this case, the eating patterns should be adjusted, for example, by eating healthy and nutritious food several times with sufficient portions. It is also important to pay attention to the quality of the food consumption for mother and baby and not just the quantity. For mothers who experience gastrointestinal problems, the need to get as much nutrition as expected becomes more obstructed. Given their nutrition intake is hampered, mothers should be more aware of the nutrition they consume from the variety of foods they eat to ensure that the nutrients for the mother and baby's requirements are met based on the doctor/nutritionist recommendations.

Pregnant women may be more susceptible to nausea, vomiting, constipation, heartburn, and dyspepsia due to the anatomic and physiologic changes. These symptoms require changes in dietary habits and lifestyles. Pregnant women may also have aversions to previously enjoyed foods. They are reluctant to eat foods with a strong smell produced by cooking or salad dressing. They usually prefer cold foods to hot foods. A healthy diet is important for pregnant women and the baby. Daily energy and essential nutrient requirements should be met during pregnancy. Women with gastrointestinal symptoms are more likely to have poor nutritional quality or poor dietary habits.

6.3. Medications and Supplements

A huge focus of attention over the past couple of years has been the use of folic acid in pregnancy. This water-soluble B-vitamin is well recognized for its role in preventing birth defects and has become the "poster vitamin" for prenatal health and development. Evidence from several studies suggests that folic acid may be effective in relieving GI disorders, such as vomiting. How closely to minimum daily stress supplement is unclear. A Norwegian study suggested that folic acid in doses as high as 5,000 mg per day has no added adverse effects over 0.6 g per day, which is the dose recommended for pregnant women at risk of neural tube defects. Other treatment options for GI symptoms during pregnancy - such as changes in diet, advice from a nurse, and suggestions of ginger, plus vitamins and minerals including vitamin B6 and calcium - do not have consistently good evidence that they help and can worsen vomiting in some women. While significant and reliable evidence involving cimetidine, glucocorticosteroids, DNS of histamine, monoaminergic agents, and antihistamines is absent, 20 mg/d of vitamin B6 and 300 mg/d of calcium might provide some efficacy when incorporated, as the update of pharmacotherapy procedures for females during pregnancy - detailed in the Cochrane Syst Review. It was noted, however, that if the minimum level of evidence is available. Research indicates that, at minimum, overall, no direct adverse effects on the unborn child or infant are created by the use of SSRI medication for the treatment of nausea and changes. Prior to the finalization of a diagnostic evaluation, dietary advice and home treatment are suggested. Conditions that would necessitate seeking medical advice would include dehydration, palpation, severe typical symptoms or unconsciousness, a decline in fetal exercise, and non-passing stool for many days.

Nevertheless, safety data for medications and supplements taken by pregnant women are collected and assessed by numerous agencies globally, such as the Centers for Disease Control and Prevention in the US, the Australian Department of Health and Ageing, the Teratology Information Services in the UK, Motherisk in Canada, and the European Network of Teratology Information Services. Their data sources include registry-based data, prospective pregnancy cohorts, and surveillance systems, and the range of GI topics covered is from acid-related disease medication to the role of folic acid in managing nausea or vomiting. Such analyses can provide initial insights into the efficacy as well as potential negative effects of therapies used by pregnant women for mild to moderate GI symptoms. This information may be useful in providing some support about the use of medications and supplements in general. However, these analyses exclude many medications used in the management of GI disorders and symptoms as well as their use for the management of more severe GI symptoms. In many cases, including the drugs used to manage more severe symptoms, new research and/or clinical guidelines are needed. Restricting medications to pregnant women may be especially important. For example, based on current data, proton-pump inhibitors and H2-receptor antagonists may cause side effects in women, including the fetus and newborn.

For most drugs and supplements, insufficient evidence exists regarding the benefits and risks of their use for managing GI symptoms during pregnancy. Hence, to help women manage these conditions effectively with a favorable benefit/risk balance, evidence-based guidance is currently limited. Furthermore, other than cautioning women to use medications as minimally as possible during pregnancy, the US FDA and Health Canada do not currently provide clear guidance on the use of medications for GI symptoms during pregnancy. This is largely because most medications have been insufficiently studied in pregnant women and so no clear understanding of their benefit/risk profile can be ascertained.

7. When to Seek Medical Attention for Gastrointestinal Symptoms During Pregnancy

There are many different gastrointestinal issues that can arise during pregnancy. Fortunately, many can be managed at home. If women display one or more of the signs described in this paper, contact a healthcare professional to discuss their symptoms. If you are pregnant, make sure that your obstetrician is informed right away. Keep your own future in mind! You are the most important caretaker for your child, and it is crucial to keep the health of both you and your baby in mind. Do not use any medications without first consulting your prescriber, as some medications have been linked to birth defects (teratogenesis). Preventing unplanned pregnancies can have a lasting effect on your health by allowing you to work with your prescriber to plan the proper treatment.

Conclusion

The following symptoms, many of which are described as concerning above, may also be warning signs indicating whether the doctor should be seen or contacted. For example, if lower back pain is present, amniotic fluid might be leaking, or if fever, vaginal discharge that has changed, or bleeding from the vagina, doctor evaluation is presumably necessary. When other conditions might be responsible for some or all of the symptoms, early treatment is likely to be the best option.

- Severe symptoms such as severe vomiting, diarrhea, cramping, or abdominal pain, or if signs of dehydration are present, may warrant medical attention. - If women suspect that early labor is underway or if they are experiencing vaginal bleeding, a doctor should evaluate them. - If the expectant mother has been diagnosed with a medical condition that can affect the intestines and cause symptoms similar to the above, immediate medical guidance might also be advisable. - Finally, if a previously pregnant woman is now nursing and taking medications, she might need to consult with a doctor for advice about her symptoms and medications before taking them.

There are several concerning symptoms that could arise during pregnancy, which might require a doctor's immediate attention. These might include:

When to seek medical attention

8. Conclusion and Summary of Key Points

Gastrointestinal symptoms are commonplace in pregnancy, which may cause some overlap of presentation with normal physiology. Both hormonal influences and anatomical changes develop during pregnancy and have been associated with clearer symptoms in previous research. Most symptoms are self-reported during history-taking and only require additional resources and diagnostic studies in women with excretion following non-invasive treatment. However, the exclusion of a change from the norm, such as the investigation of anemia in constipated women or acid suppressive therapy, who do not follow up with symptom resolution, for the menstrual bleeding during pregnancy do include invasive fiberoptic imaging. In contrast to dyspepsia associated with pregnancy, comprehensive discussion of the presentation of gastrointestinal symptoms that cause a majority of women to seek care during their pregnancy has not been described in current publications.

This review specifically outlines common symptoms women may experience during pregnancy. Symptoms such as heartburn, bloating, constipation, and hemorrhoids are thought to provoke visits to various providers, including primary care, internal medicine, obstetrics/gynecology, and gastroenterology. Often symptoms are considered physiological in nature, and in the case of fiberoptic imaging for evaluation, the process can be considered invasive and is generally avoided. Yet when taken together with chronic conditions, certain symptoms may be considered more damaging to a pregnant woman with the correlation of physiological changes, which could interfere with management of chronic conditions. Fiberoptic imaging studies can also be cumbersome for the provider due to logistical constraints. In these cases, advanced assessment and non-fiberoptic imaging studies should still be considered carefully rather than immediately following conventional treatment algorithms.

Gastrointestinal Symptoms During Pregnancy: A Comprehensive Guide

1. Introduction to Gastrointestinal Symptoms in Pregnancy

Gastrointestinal and hepatobiliary symptoms are common during gestation. They are challenging not just for patients but also for obstetricians, midwives, and primary care physicians. Certain steps, such as ranking the differential diagnosis from severe to "normal" based on patient symptoms, are necessary to alleviate and counsel an individual affected by certain symptoms. These symptoms are further coupled with emotional or psychological desperation, as many pregnant women in developing countries are poor and financially unable to communicate this to healthcare-seeking practitioners. To deal with this immense workload and concept, we tried to describe certain gastrointestinal and hepatic-biliary problems in antenatal care. With each condition, etiopathogenesis, presentation, diagnosis or investigations, and management are highlighted. This is all based on current evidence available worldwide. Moreover, special emphasis is given to a certain category as to how it impacts pregnancy and fetal health.

This chapter attempts to provide a comprehensive guide to managing gastrointestinal symptoms during gestation. The aim is not only to highlight common problems along with their management strategies but also to assist readers in ranking differential diagnoses according to the severity of symptoms. Perhaps it is most informative and practical for a vast majority of "non-specialists/specialists" who provide healthcare to women worldwide, mostly those from low-to-medium-resourced countries. It is important to acknowledge that high-resource countries have a vast pool of technological advances, interventions, and specifically trained personnel to tackle each differential diagnosis. Countries that are not so enriched with expertise, local technical advancement, interventions, and alternative support systems usually require generalized multi-faceted healthcare delivery.

2. Physiological Changes in the Gastrointestinal Tract During Pregnancy

During pregnancy, the hormonal milieu is profoundly different compared to that in non-pregnant women. Two major hormonal changes occur during pregnancy: a significant increase in estrogen and the highest levels of progesterone, then increasing almost 20-fold at delivery. In total, the increase in estrogens is 1000-fold higher than that in non-pregnant subjects. After impregnation, the increase of estrogens, together with other molecules, such as relaxin, have an interest in the relaxant effects on multiple tissues, including the muscles of the pelvic area, which are determinant in delivery and parturition. Esophageal and gastric motility are reduced, and the tone and volume of the LES are decreased in pregnancy, with an increase in the number of transient LOS relaxations (TLOSRs). The impairment of the barrier function of the lower esophagus can be correlated with the severity of symptoms during pregnancy. Increased gallbladder volume, affected emptying, and gallbladder stasis are secondary to progesterone. Stomach motility is reduced, and the decrease in antral pressure can affect gastric emptying time and drug absorption. The motility of the colon is reduced, and clinical aspects are often due to the tablet compression caused by the gravid uterus in the pelvis, but this is transient, and it quickly reverts to normal after delivery. Furthermore, lower levels of serum nitric oxide (NO) were found in pregnant compared to non-pregnant age-matched women. NO plays a critical role as a neurotransmitter in the regulation of gastrointestinal (GI) motility, and it participates in the normal control of the pregnant ileum. In early labor, the rise of NO has been suggested as a marker for pregnancy scheduling.

Pregnancy is associated with diverse physiological changes in the body. Some of these changes are pertinent to the gastrointestinal tract, and they can significantly affect the daily life of pregnant women. Many hormones, including sex steroids, and other molecules are gender-dimorphic and can play physiological and pathogenic roles in multiple tissues, including the gastrointestinal tract. Fluctuations of estrogens and progesterone related to the menstrual cycle, the luteal phase, or the contraception-mediator cycle determine significant cyclical changes such as acid-related functions and colon transit time, nausea and vomiting, bloating, and abdominal discomfort in women.

3. Common Gastrointestinal Symptoms and Their Causes

Though rarely nonphysiologic GI abnormalities, person-general, surgery-specific, or organ-imaging studies may indicate a more dangerous pathology and/or the necessity of obstetric intervention. By understanding the often-described physiologic causes of most symptoms, steps may be taken to avoid such GI afflictions.

The most common gastrointestinal complaints of pregnancy include: - Nausea and vomiting - Pyrosis (heartburn) - Constipation - Diarrhea - Abdominal pain and cramping - Hemorrhoids - Gallbladder disease - Hepatic disease

Though it may feel as though their baby's foot is constantly lodged into their stomach lining and morning sickness with retching and vomiting may be a daily, if not hourly, occurrence, pregnant persons do not suffer from gastrointestinal conditions. They deal with gastrointestinal symptoms of and caused by the altered gravid state of pregnancy. A review of the gastrointestinal system and its accompanying symptoms is indispensable in the holistic approach to pregnant patients commonly encountered in obstetrics. It also contributes to less empathetic, purely physical examination and findings among patients claiming GI symptoms without signs.

4. Nausea and Vomiting

Nausea and vomiting during pregnancy can be experienced at different times throughout gestation; it is typically more severe earlier in gestation and resolves as pregnancy progresses. The mechanisms that contribute to the symptoms of nausea and vomiting are likely multifactorial systems discussed in greater detail elsewhere in this series. Approximately 8% of women report having severe nausea without vomiting, and an additional 36% report severe nausea and vomiting. Notably, the severity of nausea and vomiting is correlated with symptom persistence, impacting maternal well-being into the third trimester. Nausea and vomiting during pregnancy are commonly associated with odors, food, and increased acidity leading to an increase in reflux-related symptoms. Gastrointestinal emptying and a subset of the symptoms of irritable bowel syndrome are experienced more frequently during pregnancy, and the review in this series provides more detail on the impact of gestation on these symptoms. Management is similar for these related problems.

Nausea and vomiting during pregnancy are common pregnancy-related symptoms. Nausea and vomiting are often referred to as 'morning sickness,' reflecting the most common time that they occur. A landmark study exemplifies the multifactorial origins of 'morning sickness,' where multiple systems covered in this series will be straw hats that contribute to nausea and vomiting during gestation. Cognitive factors, including ambivalence towards the pregnancy, most notably 'conditional love,' existed in just over half of the women who could conceive children in a follow-up study. Follow-up surveys find that many pregnant women report high levels of stress and anxiety. Before conception or in planned pregnancies, psychosocial stress such as hating the thought of being pregnant, socioeconomic status, smoking, and alcohol use can contribute to morning sickness symptoms.

5. Heartburn and Acid Reflux

Heartburn and acid reflux can be treated or managed in several ways. A good place to start is to identify and avoid foods that trigger these symptoms – in general, these are spicy, fatty, fried or acidic food and drink. Eating smaller meals and cutting down on drinks high in caffeine or alcohol can also help to keep these symptoms at bay. In bed, it can be helpful to elevate your head using an extra pillow as this reduces the amount of acid that travels to your esophagus during the night. Gaviscon (an alginate that floats straight back down the esophagus without side effects) can be a good addition to this, as it forms a physical barrier on top of the stomach contents. Ranitidine, a pregnancy-safe medication, can be used to reduce the amount of stomach acid your body produces. Some gynecologists have the policy to combine ranitidine with Gaviscon for an improved effect.

Heartburn and acid reflux go hand in hand for many women, with a prevalence of 90% during pregnancy. Although the exact cause is unknown, the increasing levels of progesterone during pregnancy are thought to play a role. They relax the muscles around the entrance to the stomach, allowing stomach acid to leak back up into the esophagus, resulting in the painful, burning feeling known as heartburn. The symptoms of heartburn/acid reflux curse many women, especially after eating, when lying down or slouching. Severe episodes can lead to regurgitation and stomach acid in the mouth. Acid reflux doesn't come without its discomfort, with many experiencing nausea and fatigue as a result. Like most pregnancy symptoms, heartburn typically worsens in the third trimester when the baby is at its largest, and the symptoms are more pronounced when lying down with gravity aiding the acid to travel upwards.

6. Constipation

To help alleviate constipation during pregnancy, pregnant individuals should increase their intake of fiber but be sure to do so gradually in order to prevent gas and bloating. Fruit, vegetables, and whole grains in particular are good sources of fiber. They should also drink six to eight glasses of fluids, especially water, a day and engage in regular exercise, which can help alleviate gastrointestinal symptoms in general. If positivity can be reframed and constipation is viewed as the body's coping mechanism to reduce fetal exposure to chemicals, pregnant individuals will find it much easier to tolerate. For pregnant women who continue to struggle with constipation, the following can also be considered: Increasing intake of natural yogurt to help improve gut microbiome balance, although scientific evidence is still in progress. All food that is high in prunes may also help reduce levels of constipation. Opting for foods and drinks that are rich in prebiotics, which help promote good bacteria in the gut, often show some benefits as the gut adjusts during pregnancy. If trying prebiotic supplements, it is important to start on a low dose and gradually increase.

Constipation is extremely common during pregnancy. It affects up to fifty-six percent of pregnant women, especially during the first and third trimesters. Individuals' colons slow down during pregnancy. The hormone progesterone causes smooth muscle fibers, i.e. simple and multinucleated cells that allow muscles to contract, in the body to relax. This relaxation allows the uterus to expand during pregnancy, but it also causes the bowel muscles to contract less frequently and may lead to constipation. The growing uterus can lead to constipation. It compresses the intestines, essentially squeezing the poop through a smaller space which can prevent normal stool passage. The growing uterus also lowers the amount of liquid found in the stool, further hardening it.

7. Diarrhea

- Eat small, frequent meals throughout the day instead of three large meals. All GI symptoms are more prevalent in women who skip meals. - Drink water or carbohydrate/electrolyte-containing beverages with meals. - Limit caffeine-containing beverages, spicy, and gas-producing foods and agents, alcohol, and dairy if lactose intolerant.

7.5 Prevention

Diarrhea has been reported by between 7-9% of US pregnant women. In Colombia and a Paraguayan Border Clinic serving women who access prenatal care in both Brazil and Paraguay, diarrhea during pregnancy and the postpartum is experienced by as many as 1 in 3 pregnant women. Women who have a reported GI disorder, such as inflammatory bowel disease (as in clinical setting studies cited above), while pregnant, reportedly experience symptoms such as diarrhea and other GI-related discomfort less frequently, possibly due to increased knowledge about the topic. In Colombian pregnant women presenting to a hospital with abdominal pain (otherwise not specified as being GI-pain) during pregnancy and the postpartum period, diarrhea was one of many causes of pain and reported infrequently.

7.4 Impact on Maternal Well-Being

The development of diarrhea during pregnancy is multifactorial and may be related to a wide array of local (e.g., gut bacteria), systemic, and drug-induced changes (e.g., diarrhea-promoting iron supplementation, antibiotics) taking place during pregnancy. The marked changes in gastrointestinal (GI) motility, gastric emptying, and increased water and electrolyte reabsorption via the kidneys and the colon—leading to mild dehydration (discussed in Management)—together with the broad changes in the gut microbiome that pregnant women experience, are proposed mechanisms. The changing gut microbiome of pregnant women also changes the way they process the sugars from fruits, vegetables, and grains, which may have some relevance for diarrhea during pregnancy. GI-related infections and pre-existing disorders which may lead to diarrhea prior to pregnancy, such as celiac disease, irritable bowel disease, or inflammatory bowel disease, are reportedly positively associated with the occurrence of diarrhea during pregnancy.

7.3 Causes

During pregnancy, diarrhea has been reported by around 8% of pregnant women in the United States. It is listed among the top disorders diagnosed during pregnancy. Episodes of diarrhea extend from the second trimester until the postpartum period in around one-third of pregnant women affected by diarrhea.

7.2 Prevalence

Diarrhea is the passage of three or more loose, watery, or liquid stools per day. Acute diarrhea typically lasts less than 14 days, while diarrhea is considered chronic when it persists for at least four weeks. The World Health Organization (WHO) has defined the term "mother-baby pair affected by one or more episodes" of "acutely malnourishing diarrhea" as two or more loose stools per day in a child (child does not ingest normal amounts of food for more than a few days with a change in the child's accommodation, health care seeking, or preparation of meals, or the presence of any of the following: black stool indicating digested blood, other stool indicating visible blood, or visible mucus.

7.1 Definition

8. Abdominal Pain and Cramping

While passing gas can diminish the discomfort, belly pain and cramping during pregnancy can also be a sign of severe medical problems, such as placental abruption, that require urgent evaluation. If accompanied by vaginal bleeding, this kind of severe pain can indicate this kind of risk. In pregnant women, appendicitis can also be tricky to identify because the inflammation can be in a different position. That's why, because of the chance of preterm birth, many surgeons would prefer to act on appendicitis during pregnancy and perform a Caesarean section if necessary at the same time. Women experiencing stomach cramps and pains should consult their healthcare provider if these last any length of discomfort. If the stomach pain doesn't go away when the cramps disappear or gets worse, seeking help is necessary.

During pregnancy, the release of certain hormones may cause the walls of the bowels to relax, slowing down the digestive process. This can cause mild pain and cramping, similar to the discomfort experienced during menstruation. Normal uterine growth can also result in mild abdominal discomfort. There are other things that can show up as abdominal discomfort that during pregnancy could be more concerning. False labor, or Braxton-Hicks contractions, can present as intense pain. During this period, short and mild uterine muscle contractions happen with increasing frequency. Despite the discomfort during this procedure, Braxton-Hicks contractions do not cause cervical thinning or dilation, a mark of labor. Also, severe intestinal gas pain may appear.

9. Hemorrhoids

Signs and symptoms: Pregnant patients report symptoms due to the effect of hemorrhoids on their quality of life. This condition frequently causes discomfort, bleeding, and pain in these patients. Most problems center around prolapse and a frequency of prolapse. Pregnant patients may report acute severe thrombotic pain or symptoms of a chronic ache. The affected women avoid bulging, defecation, sitting, standing, walking, squatting, or sleeping with a straight leg. In the field of nonoperative methods for the treatment of hemorrhoids, conservative measures such as diet improvement (intake of dietary fiber, water consumption), adopting good toilet habits (avoid harsh wiping or scrubbing, applying moistened towelettes to the affected area, avoidance of analgesic-containing products application, avoidance of suppositories containing vasoconstrictors and compliance with the natural urge of defecation) and encouragement of physical activity should be advised to alleviate the symptoms and improve the quality of life for pregnant patients. Prevention is better than the cure. Pregnant patients should be referred to a dietician and referred to a physiotherapist for physical function and myofascial pelvic floor muscle relaxation evaluation and training, in order to apply preventive strategies to address hemorrhoids and other lower gastrointestinal symptoms. Management of hemorrhoids should be mainly conservative.

Causes and associations: The main factors that contribute to hemorrhoids in pregnant patients are the pressure from the fetus during pregnancy and childbirth, hormonal changes, increased abdominal pressure due to constipation, and hormone increase. The occurrence of constipation aggravates the risk of hemorrhoids. In patients who have never reported symptoms of hemorrhoids, increased body mass index, repeated pregnancy, and constipation are risk factors for this disorder.

Occurrence in pregnant patients: Hemorrhoids are a common problem during pregnancy. It is estimated that the fetus carries an increased risk of hemorrhoids; this occurs in approximately 85% of women who complete childbirth. Nevertheless, the first symptoms during pregnancy are reported to a greater extent in late months of pregnancy and in labor.

10. Gallbladder Issues

Despite the general incidence numbers, for a woman who is pregnant, their incidence will range greatly based on particular characteristics including those which include race, body mass index (BMI) and more. Studies have shown that the prevalence of gallstone disease during pregnancy is much greater in women with a higher BMI. If a woman possesses any symptoms of cholelithiasis or gallstones at the time of pregnancy, there could be an increased risk for gallstone-associated complications such as acute cholecystitis, choledocholithiasis, and acute pancreatitis. At times, the discomfort of gallbladder distress can radiate to the shoulder area and lie between the shoulder blades. Concerns for specific cases associated with choledocholithiasis can develop when the gallstone migrates from the gallbladder to the common bile duct (CBD), and occurs in 10% of women with gallstone symptoms during pregnancy. Identifying if women are experiencing choledocholithiasis in the presence of pain and other symptoms is important from a management standpoint for further moving patients along the continuum of care. If the gallbladder is the source of pain, from a cholelithiasis standpoint, then management is somewhat different. Scoring systems exist for determining treatment options, and most clinicians use the Tokyo Guidelines to determine patients who are able to await routine surgery after treatment with analgesics and antibiotics. The conundrum of what to do with a woman who presents with imaging findings of ACT but total bilirubin levels less than 1.8 is debatable. Superimposed gallstone pancreatitis on pancreatitis is extremely high during pregnancy as well. Pancreatitis scores can also be utilized for determining evidence of acute necrotizing pancreatitis on imaging, and also for determining treatment options. Normally a woman will improve with supportive care alone. For those cases with gallstone pancreatitis, ERCP is not advised and is higher on the list of options after the patient has delivered.

The most common reason for gallbladder diagnoses during pregnancy is cholelithiasis. There are generally higher cholesterol saturation and a low ejection fraction for the gallbladder during pregnancy beginning at the first trimester, and these percentages continue to increase until delivery. Decreased gallbladder motility and increased cholesterol excretion in bile are some of the consequences from changes in metabolic hormones such as estrogen during pregnancy. The development of gallstones in the gallbladder is due to cholesterol crystal formation, which comes from supersaturated bile, and poor functioning of the gallbladder to empty bile. Inflammation of the gallbladder, and even potential gallstone obstruction of the common bile duct, can be caused by the physical presence of the gallstones. In cholelithiasis, this can cause pain and potential pancreatitis. The elucidation of the imaging diagnosis by history and physical is the next step guiding the treatment options.

11. Management and Treatment of Gastrointestinal Symptoms

1. Management of nausea and vomiting during pregnancy: a resource widely yet too often summarized as "avoid spicy foods, eat small, frequent meals, and consider ginger and vitamin B6". The management summary includes 39 points on dietary and lifestyle modifications, 10 over-the-counter medications, 12 prescription medications, and 16 preventive strategies. 2. Management of heartburn and upper abdominal pain during pregnancy: not only a systemic summary of prevention by avoiding a fatty diet and cigarette smoke but a comprehensive overview. Our heartburn management summary includes 29 points on lifestyle and dietary modifications, 6 over-the-counter medications, 2 prescription medications, and 20 preventive strategies. 3. Upper abdominal pain management in pregnant individuals. We provide dietary and lifestyle modifications and different pain management guidelines for gallbladder and non-gallbladder pain. Our upper abdominal pain summary includes 9 points on dietary and lifestyle recommendations, and 14 over-the-counter medications that are recognized as safe to use.

For each of the gastrointestinal (GI) symptoms discussed in this handbook, we provide a section with comprehensive guidance on the management and treatment of these symptoms. Management and treatment recommendations often involve lifestyle and dietary modifications, which constitute the mainstay of treatment during pregnancy. We provide these recommendations not only for pregnant individuals but also for non-pregnant individuals and therefore do not provide medications that are unsafe for pregnancy. For medications that are considered safe to use during pregnancy based on FDA guidelines, we also offer treatment options with over-the-counter and prescription medications. Where available and relevant, we offer preventive strategies for managing GI symptoms.

12. Dietary and Lifestyle Modifications

Increased risk of nausea and vomiting: Location of flatus and release of stool are regulated by the position and strength of the pelvic floor muscles; this position is assisted by sitting. Sitting with the posterior pelvis further forward than the ischial tuberosities relaxes the pelvic floor to allow easier defecation. Active forward leaning can further facilitate this interaction, as it tightens the abdominal wall and results in an increased pressure differential in favor of stool expulsion. Giving birth in this squatting position has been shown to be associated with a shorter second stage of labor. Further research on the benefit of delivering in a squat position is warranted, especially considering an ongoing cesarean delivery epidemic.

Increased risk of diarrhea, constipation, and heartburn: Patients may maximize nutrition by taking advantage of their appetite, while keeping these symptoms to a minimum. It is vital to encourage these patients to consume a high fiber diet and to remain well hydrated. Furthermore, encouraging patients to partake in light physical exercise as directed by the obstetrician may keep abdominal complaints to a minimum as well.

Dietary and lifestyle modifications: There are ways to make dietary and lifestyle changes in order to manage gastrointestinal discomfort during pregnancy. The following are some simple modifications women can make to ease various symptoms. In general, promoting safe, thoroughly cooked meals, refreshing snacks, and plenty of water are always recommended.

13. Over-the-Counter Medications

Mylanta, Maalox, Rolaids, and Tums are all OTC antacids that are safe to take when pregnant and can be used to help reduce heartburn and GERD symptoms. Over-the-counter omeprazole is the preferred treatment plan for severe heartburn and GERD during pregnancy. Pregnancy category B medications should be used preferentially. However, if those are not satisfactory, the use of pregnancy category C medications for a short period of time may be considered based on the risk versus benefit ratio discussed by the healthcare provider. Pepcid and Zantac are both medications that are category B medications that are safe to take during pregnancy and can be used to help reduce the incidence of GERD and heartburn. Indigestion or Upset Stomach – Mylanta, Maalox, Rolaids, Tums. Some categories of gas relievers in pregnancy are limited. Bottom line: No Gas-X.

Many over-the-counter (OTC) medications are safe to use when experiencing gastrointestinal symptoms. However, all medications should be taken under the guidance of a healthcare provider and only for a short period of time. Pregnant individuals should always talk to their healthcare provider before starting a new medication. Natural options, such as ginger, may also be an option to help reduce morning sickness and GI discomfort, but should not be used by pregnant individuals with a history of miscarriage. Loperamide can be used to help manage episodes of loose stools or diarrhea, however, it is very important to make sure that pregnancy is not a factor as loperamide is a category C medication. Pregnancy category C medications should be avoided if possible, and taken only for a very short term if needed and only under the guidance of the healthcare provider.

14. Prescription Medications

Safety concerns Many medications and gastrointestinal pharmacologic agents exist which are considered safe, according to what we know now, for use by pregnant women. Some prescription drugs and treatments that are effective for the general population may not be safe for pregnant women. This does not necessarily mean that they will harm the baby, but doctors are not certain. In most instances, the U.S. Food and Drug Administration (FDA) has not given approval for the use of drugs in pregnant women because doing a study in these women would not be ethical. However, a few drugs in our list of medications here have been approved by the FDA for use in pregnancy. Some of these are for symptoms of pregnancy, such as increased nausea and vomiting. Others are drugs that have been available for other uses and have become available for treatment of other diseases or conditions during pregnancy. If a drug has been approved by the FDA, you will see this stated at the top of the page for that drug or treatment. For the most part, medications listed are at least safe in pregnancy, meaning that there is no evidence of harm. However, the decision to use any drug in pregnancy should be based on the expectant mother's symptoms and clinical history alone. Prior to using any medications, it is important that you consult with your doctor to ensure that you are using the proper medication for your specific symptoms. In summary, medications should be limited in pregnancy, and dietary and lifestyle changes should be the mainstay.

Physicians consider a number of factors before prescribing medication for pregnant women. Among these factors are the woman's overall health, how long she has been pregnant, and her age. The amount of medicine that reaches the baby depends on how soluble the drug is and how acidic the woman's urine is. This amount also depends on the way the woman's kidneys are functioning. In general, the second trimester is a period of rapid growth of the baby, which can sometimes cleanse certain medications from its system. It is not recommended to use any drug during the first trimester when the baby is forming.

15. When to Seek Medical Attention

Slow fetal growth, indicated by lack of appropriate weight gain, should be reported to the physician; addressing malnutrition can help ensure the baby's growth. Generally, GI problems are not viewed as major complications of pregnancy unless weight loss ensues or serious medical problems are identified or must be resolved with medications and possible hospitalization, frequent monitoring of the fetal heart rate or appropriate laboratory studies. Gastroenterologists, obstetricians, and primary care physicians will both tell you that most of their pregnant patients who present with GI symptoms are those with complaints that have become chronic or are part of their routine medical conditions. This is especially true if the typical measures that most pregnant women use for constipation, frequent heartburn, gallbladder problems, and other common GI challenges do not work.

The following symptoms may suggest problems that need to be addressed promptly by a physician, including red flags for serious conditions or warning signs for possible complications. Red or alarming flags include recurrent episodes, complications of symptoms, or symptoms that do not resolve. Alarming symptoms that suggest possible complications include a fever, symptoms that occur at night, inability to maintain adequate intake for greater than 24 hours, concern for dehydration, hematemesis, hematochezia (bleeding from the anus and rectum that is either bright red or maroon-colored) or melena stool (black, tarry stool), unintentional weight loss, and unremitting vomiting.

16. Impact of Gastrointestinal Symptoms on Pregnancy and Fetal Health

The occurrence of gastrointestinal diseases also has a direct impact on the development of the fetus. It is known that women whose pregnancy was complicated, for example, by chronic hyperacid gastritis carry children with reduced psychomotor development. Her child's brain is about two months behind in development compared to a child who was carried in a lower acid environment. The children of mothers with diseases or complications of the digestive system during pregnancy also have a poorer adaptive environment. Care should be taken to ensure that the causes of such diseases are diagnosed and treated on time, as delayed treatment can lead to dysfunctions and, consequently, diseases in the child. In addition, a pregnant woman who suffers from certain gastrointestinal diseases such as Helicobacter pylori or Escherichia coli gastropathies can experience, among other things, pregnancy poisoning, causing both herself and the child to have serious health problems, and skipping a meal can lead to death. Factors causing perinatal mortality. Thus, attention should be paid to a patient's complaint-treatment diagnosis. So it is very important to ensure that a comprehensive approach is taken to the diagnosis and treatment of such disorders in pregnant women or women planning pregnancy. This action will contribute, to some extent, to improving medicine and the health of society.

2. Impact of Gastrointestinal Symptoms on Pregnancy and Fetal Health

Disorders of the gastrointestinal (GI) tract are a very important factor affecting the quality of a woman's life during pregnancy. It is widely known that discomfort and pain decrease the quality of a woman's life. Therefore, early diagnosis and comprehensive treatment of such disorders are important to make a woman more likely to pursue pregnancy. They also allow her to carry a pregnancy without experiencing discomfort and pain and thus to avoid complications that could endanger her or her child. Although the effect of GI diseases on pregnancy is still little investigated and ambiguous, these relationships, to some extent, help us better understand the pathological and physiological processes that occur in pregnant women. During complications, GI diseases can lead to a pregnancy loss, premature birth, low birth rate, childbirth through abdominal cavity cut, anemia or uterine fibroids. Mothers who feel good and do not have any ailments, give birth to children with optimal weight and height, who develop and function physiologically. This reference should lead gynecologists and midwives to a more comprehensive assessment of pregnancy and delivery because a holistic postpartum approach plays an increasingly important role in the improving quality of health. Since the mother's health is associated with the child's health, a complete health assessment is necessary for both pregnancy and childbirth, but also for the baby through childbirth and after delivery.

17. Potential Complications and Risks

As the body adapts during pregnancy, certain physiological changes occur as a direct result of anatomical and hormonal influences. Nausea and vomiting, for example, have been correlated with up to a 60% decreased risk of pregnancy loss. It is commonly known and covered by every doctor who has ever taken care of a pregnant person that anesthesia is far less effective in parturients that also have heartburn and/or GERD signs and symptoms. This necessitates both the necessity of adequately managing such pain through the labor process, as well as the necessity of identifying, preventing, and treating GERD during pregnancy. Cholelithiasis and acute cholecystitis are discussed elsewhere in limited detail for obstetric medicine with severe gastroenterology conundrums.

Several potential consequences can result from untreated gastrointestinal symptoms during pregnancy. Severe vomiting can lead to metabolic alkalosis, malnutrition, and significant weight loss, including risks of esophageal or Mallory-Weiss tears. Prolonged constipation may lead to fecal impaction and mega-colon. GERD can cause Barrett's esophagus, esophageal strictures, or esophageal ulcers in the non-pregnant population. Intra-abdominal pressure from a growing uterus presents an additional risk factor when considering signs and symptoms of cholelithiasis. Left untreated, gallstone pancreatitis could lead to premature labor or fetal death. Pancreatic cancer is not typically seen in young women. Developing pregnant people commonly seek out new OB/GYN care and midwives, allowing these providers opportunities to evaluate and manage signs and symptoms of more serious gastrointestinal conditions that would not otherwise go addressed.

Complications and risks

18. Preventive Strategies

Community Resources: - Provide diet-related and physical activity support via local First Steps site or community programs. - A referral or more individualized dietary counseling may be needed.

Preventive Monitoring: - Assess at every visit for development of gastrointestinal symptoms (e.g., nausea, vomiting, heartburn, bleeding, constipation, diarrhea, gas, or bloating). - Identify and treat any nutrition-related problems earlier, before they progress to become difficult to manage.

Teaching goals: - Avoid rigorous or exercise activities that may cause stomach upset. - Encourage slow, rhythmic breathing.

Lifestyle: - Physical activity planning includes obtaining 30 min or more of moderate exercise on most, if not all, days of the week. - Perform exercises different from those done on nonpregnant days.

Teaching goals: - Choose a variety of high-fiber foods to meet recommended intake levels (e.g., breads, cereals, fruits, vegetables, or salads). - Know portion sizes for high-fiber foods. - Drink water throughout the day (ideally 6-8 glasses a day).

Nutrition: - Follow recommended weight guidelines to avoid excessive weight gain that contributes to gastroesophageal reflux and constipation. - Increase fiber and fluid intake.

19. Dr. Priya Patel's Expert Advice

What advice would you give to pregnant readers struggling with persistent constipation? Is it okay to take a stimulant laxative while pregnant? Dr. Patel says: "Most types of constipation respond well to simple lifestyle changes and diet modifications. Where symptoms are more severe or not controlled, over-the-counter laxatives may be suitable. At all times, recommendations are best made on an individual basis. However, stimulant laxatives (e.g. senna) should be avoided if possible. They remain relatively poorly absorbed in the gut and, worse, little work has been performed on pregnant people. However, less is recognized about the actual effect of accidental exposures on developing babies. Macrogols (Bio-Laxative) and lactulose are options for which better evidence is available and they are generally better first-line choices. Always talk with your GP before beginning any constipation treatments. If it looks like constipation is really serious or getting worse, book an appointment with a healthcare professional.

This essay now features expert insight from Dr. Priya Patel, an expert in treating pregnant patients with gastrointestinal symptoms. Dr. Patel provides remarkable insight into how the gastrointestinal symptoms of pregnancy may be managed. She is a specialist in obstetrics and gastrointestinal health during pregnancy and is qualified to offer advice to those experiencing digestive issues while they are pregnant and expectant mothers.

20. Frequently Asked Questions (FAQs)

3. Can dietary intervention mitigate a slow bowel migration or decrease hemorrhoids? By adding high fiber foods to one's diet, such as fruits, vegetables, juices, and high fiber cereals, one can increase the amount of weight in their stool as well as the speed of bowel movements. This decreases the urge to strain on the toilet, which can result in hemorrhoids. In addition to the aforementioned, drinking at least 6-8 cups of fluids a day can promote the digestion of high fiber foods. Some relevant sources include water, fruit juice, or clear soups.

2. When increasing one's fluid intake, what tips can patients be given? One should aim to drink one quart of fluids throughout the day, taking slow sips of liquid when thirsty. It is helpful to drink greater quantities of fluids (like milk, juice, or water) in between meals, instead of during meals. After vomiting or diarrhea has ceased, the complete volume of the mother's balanced diet will be calculated. Then, they should divide this number by two in order to establish the amount of water they should drink daily.

1. What should a pregnant person experiencing frequent vomiting or diarrhea do? This scenario results in the two potential risk factors of dehydration and malnutrition. By increasing one's fluid intake and including a low-fat diet, these symptoms can be ameliorated. Furthermore, a multivitamin may be taken to ensure proper nutrition.

21. Conclusion and Final Thoughts

Encouragement of normal bowel habits and behavior extends to the fetus as well. Anastasi and colleagues reported significantly decreased meconium staining of the amniotic fluid in mothers who took fewer opioids, which suggests not only fetal well-being but also a subjective perception of less gastrointestinal discomfort. Colace is effective in preventing postpartum constipation, a positive implication for maternal well-being postpartum. Women with abnormal gastrointestinal function experience this as a continuous symptom: helping just a little in the movements does not entirely relieve the sensation of cramping and fullness. Future research should be aimed at developing a comprehensive, systemic picture of the bowel and its function during pregnancy and the puerperium to develop anticipatory approaches to handle weird, chronic symptoms of interest to practicing professionals and researchers. In the long run, we need earlier intervention and a variable healthcare team to follow patients proactively, serving as a single source of recommendation and education as we view each patient uniquely and globally, stressing the necessity of prenatal psychological guidance. Given the well-documented influence of GI health on mom stress and vice versa, early intervention would also directly help fetus well exercise and modify future GI systems settlements.

In conclusion, pregnancy is a time when women suffer from various troubling gastrointestinal symptoms of a physiological nature. The most common symptoms are connected to motor function and changes (reflux). Diarrhea at the end of pregnancy is a warning sign, and perinatal doctors should take this into account during the women's check-ups. Women with a history of good/normal bowel movement seem to have a lower probability of developing constipation during pregnancy.